AF488668

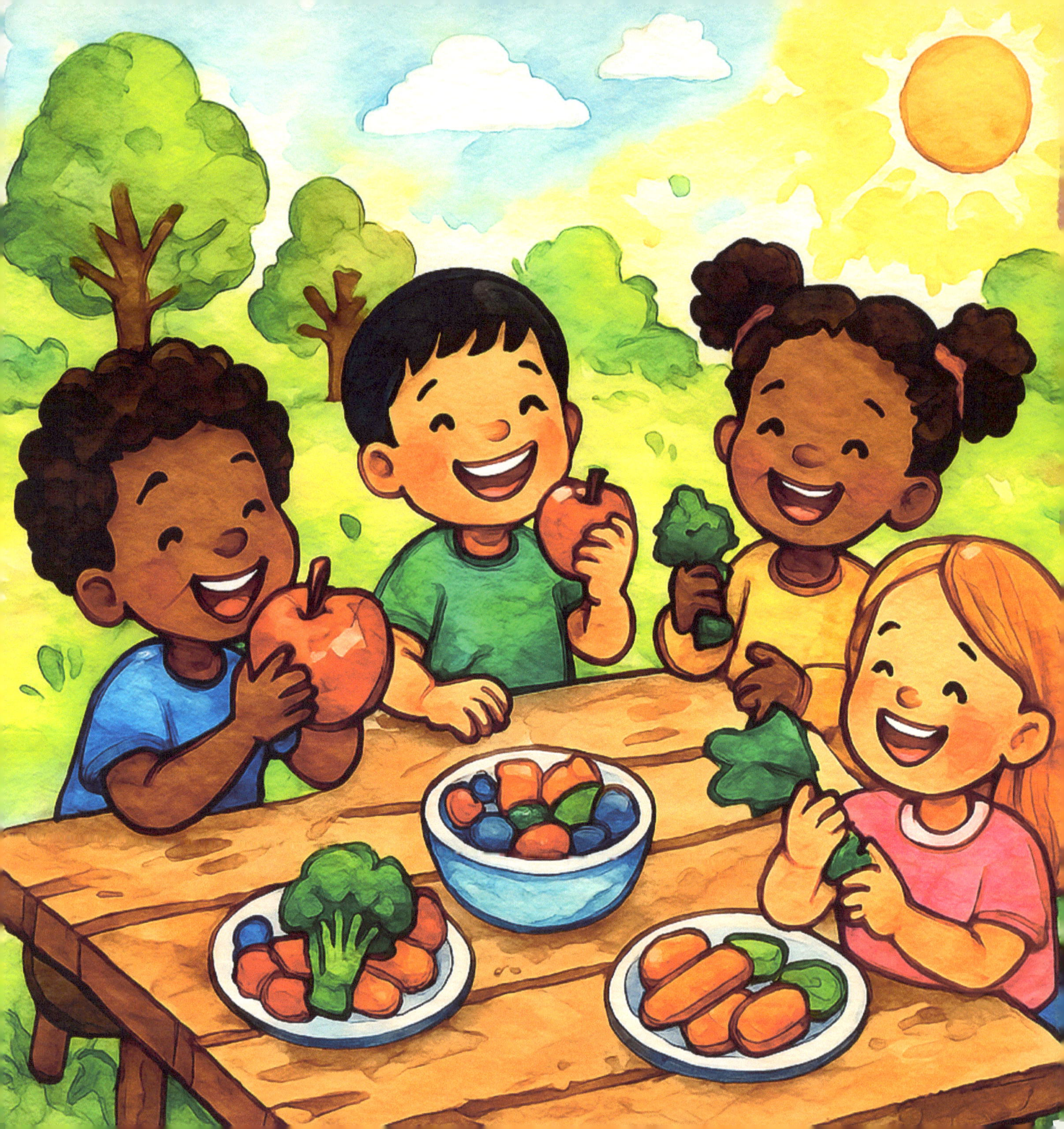

Chomp, Chomp, Chew, Chew. Fruits and veggies are good for you.

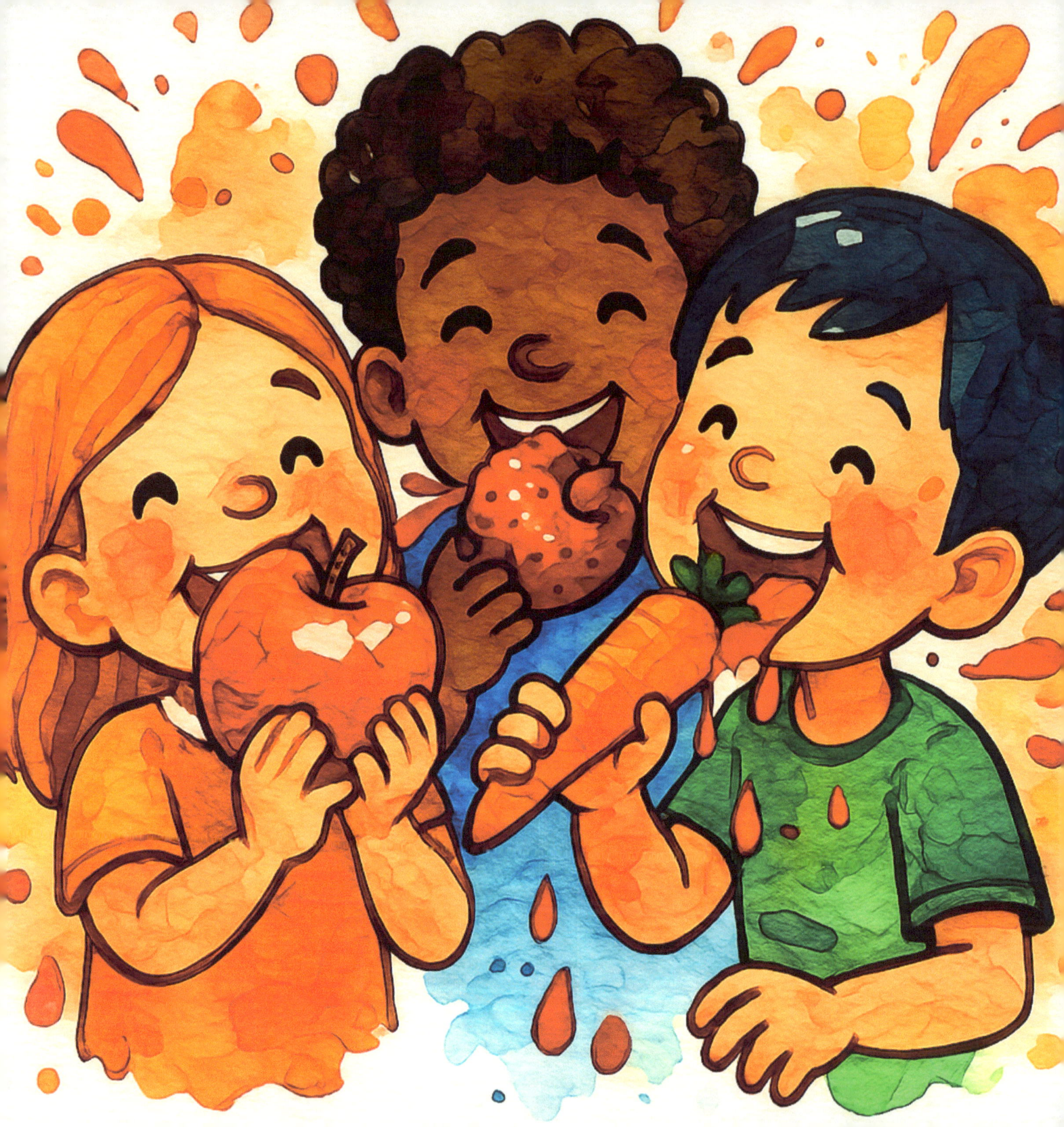

Yummy, delicious,
super nutritious.

Chomp, Chomp,
Chew, Chew.

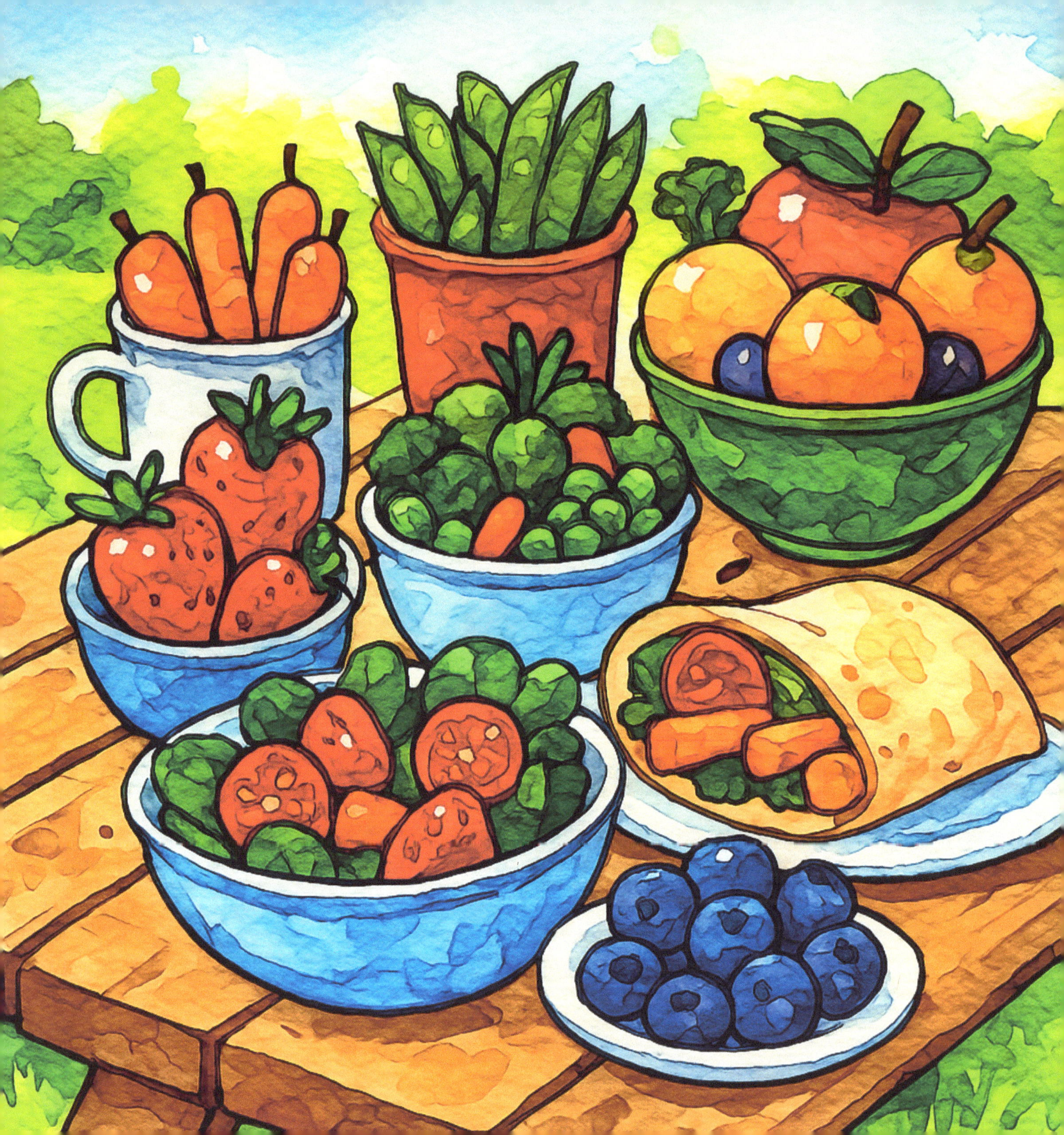

In a cup,
in a bowl,
on a plate,
on a roll.

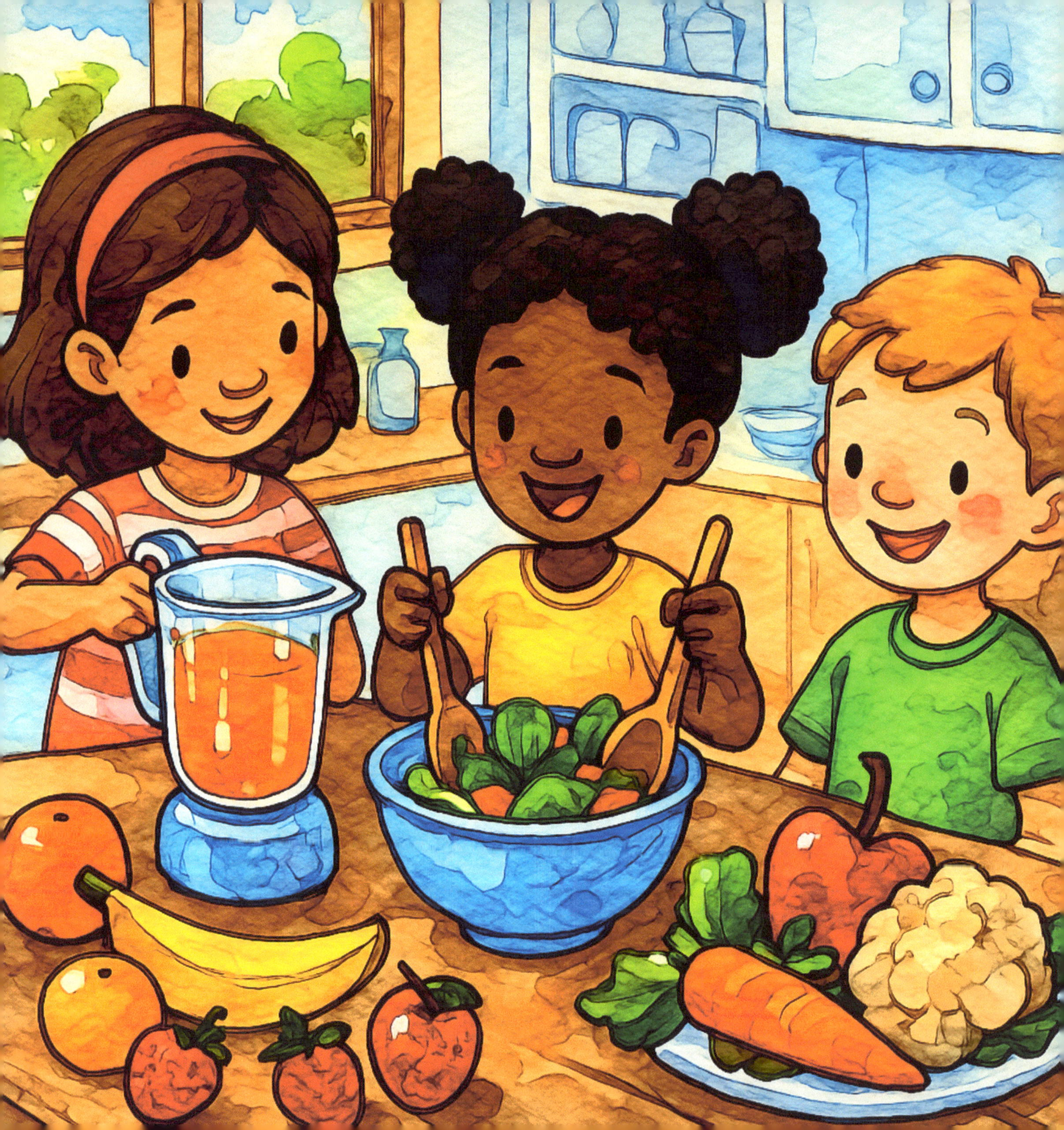

In a salad,
with all sides of dishes,
or even in smoothies,
they're just
yummy-licious.

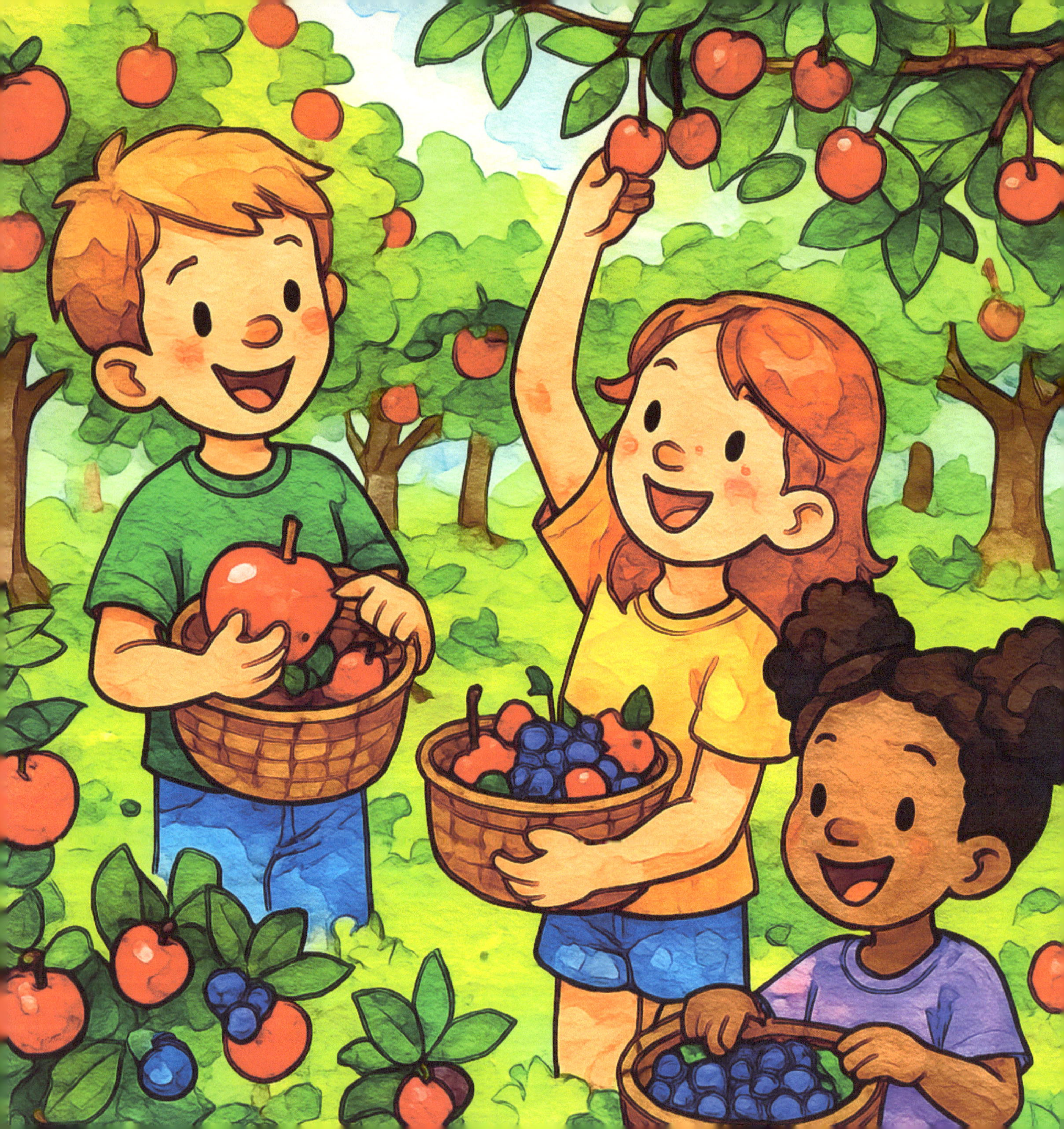

Eat some apples,
eat some berries,
try some oranges,
try some cherries.

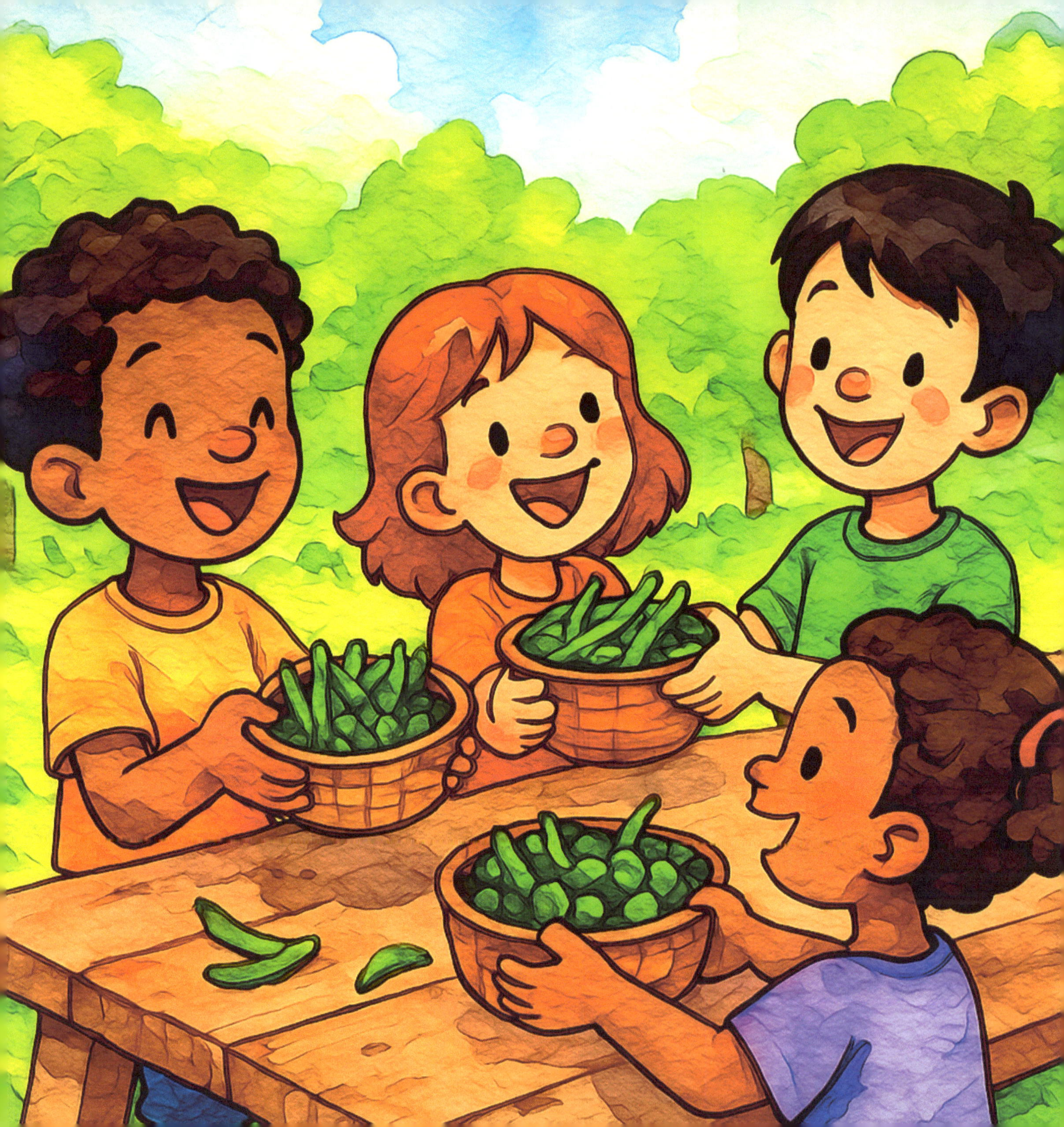

Pass some beans,
pass the peas,
they're so good —
can I have more,
please?

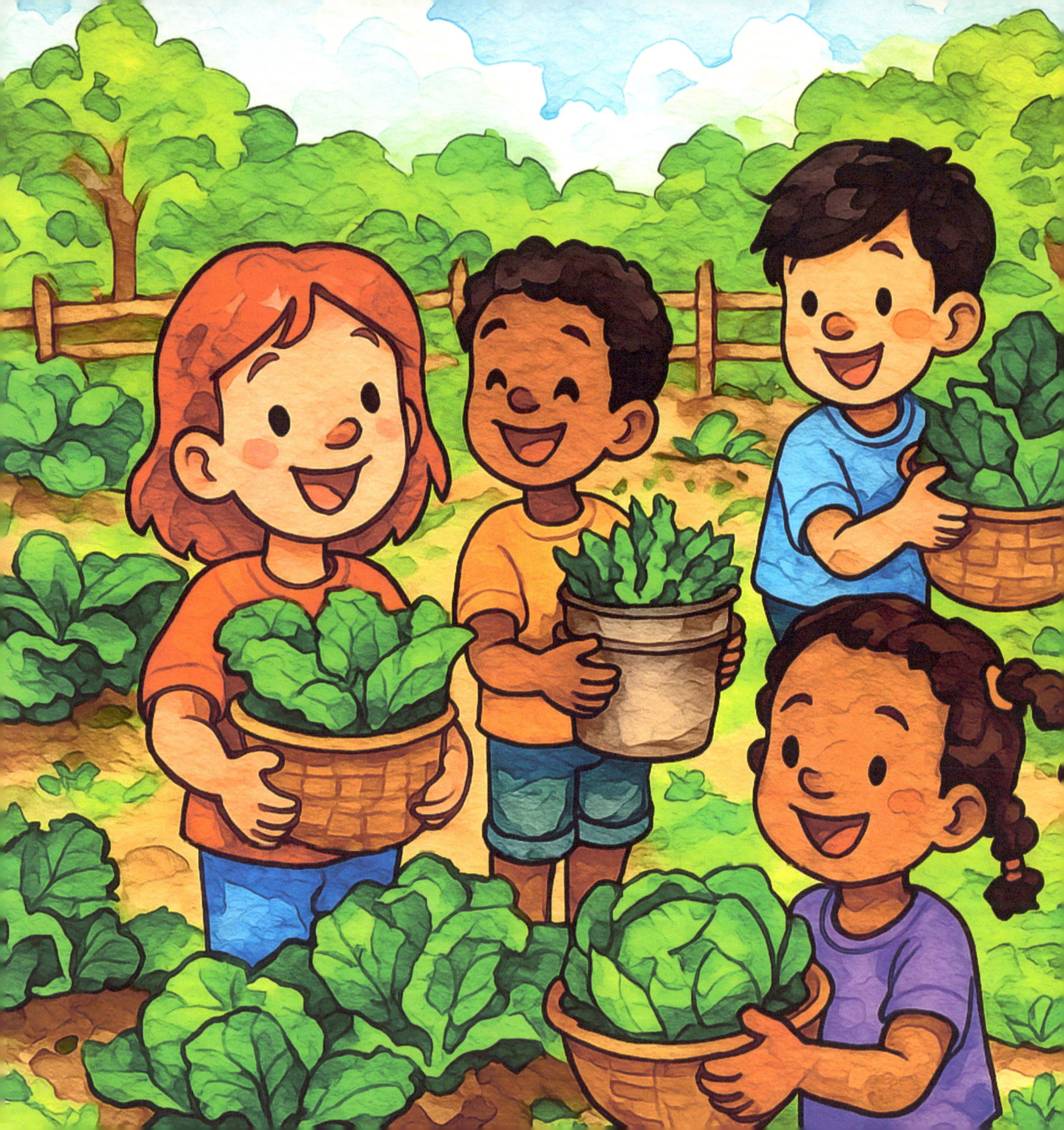

Lettuce, spinach,
cabbage, kale-
pick it by the basket,
or pick it by the pail.

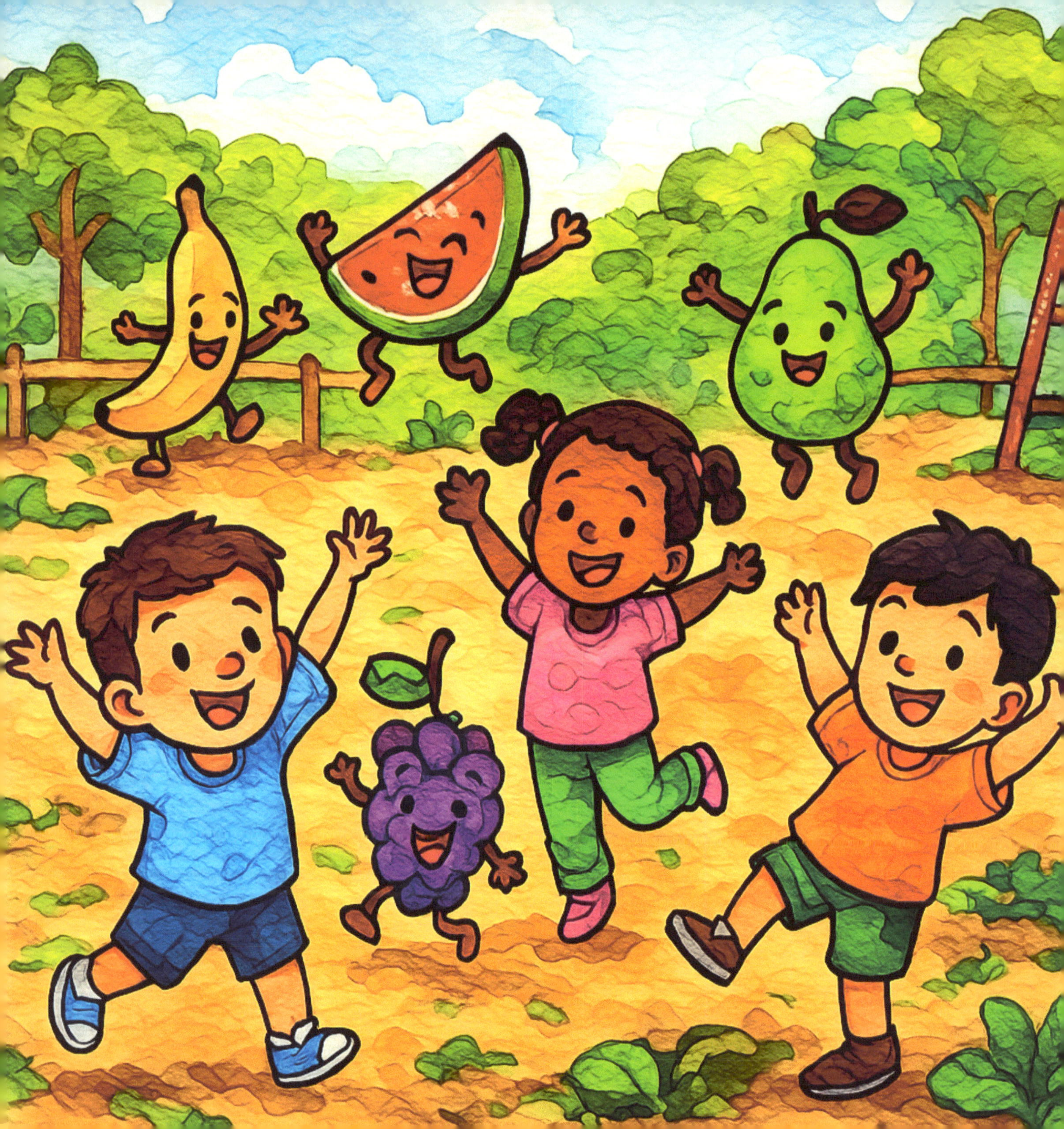

Bananas, melons, grapes, and pears- they're good for your bodies, from your toes to your hairs.

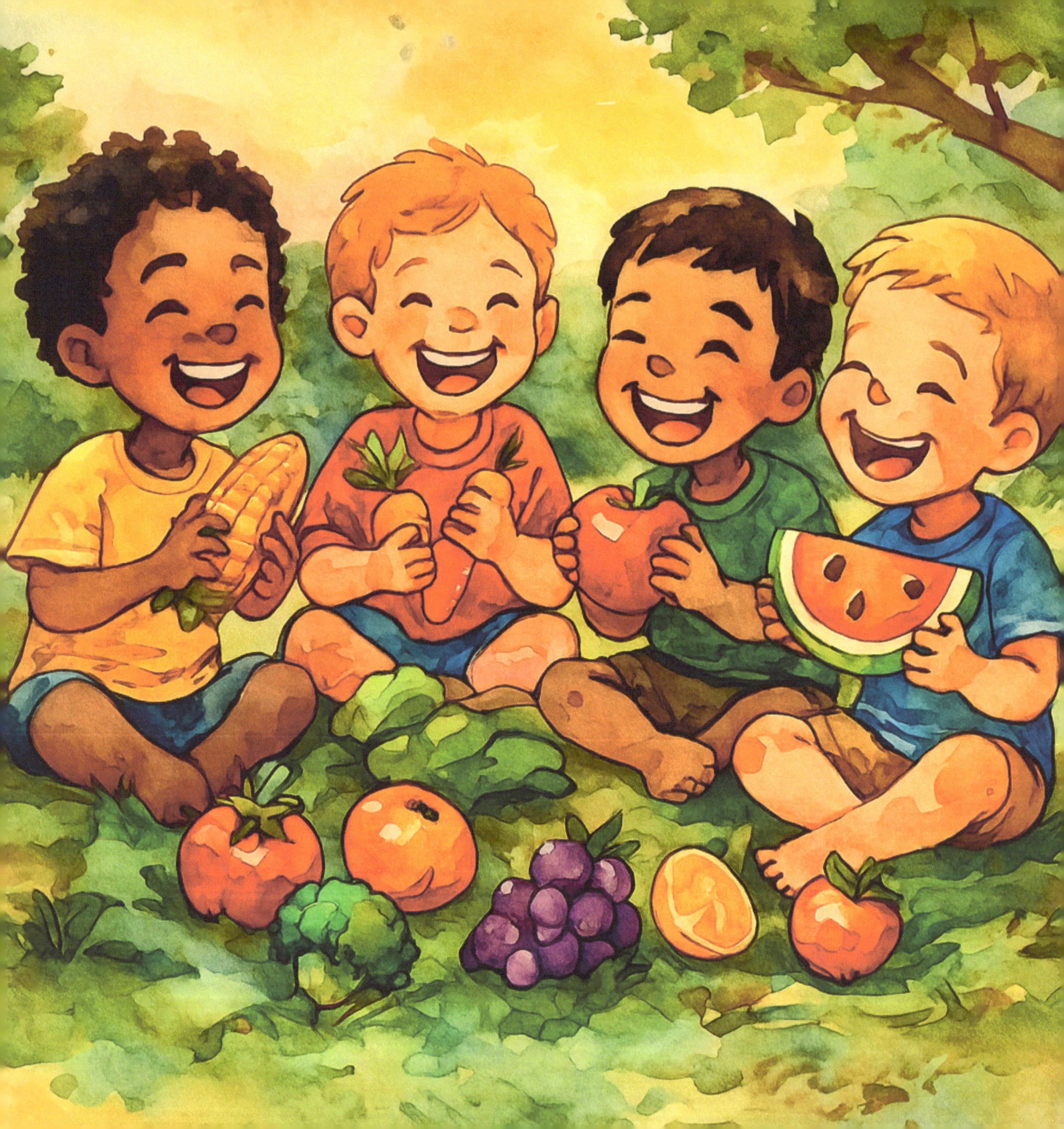

Kiwis, plums,
leafy greens,
potatoes, carrots, and
tangerines.
Fruits and veggies
are good for you.
So, Chomp, and Chomp,
and Chew, and Chew.

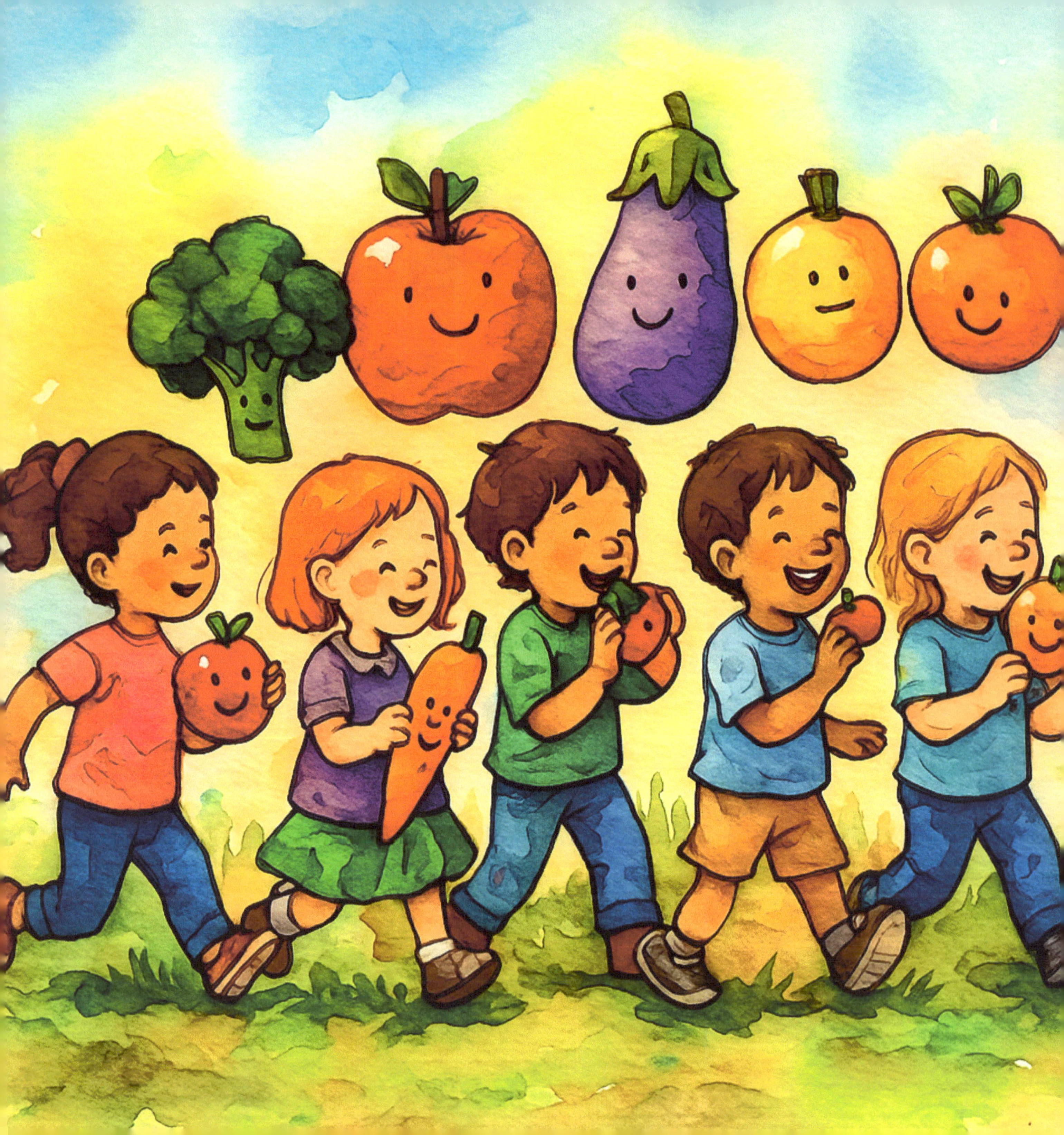

Avocados to
zucchinis,
and all letters
in betweenies.
Pass me some fruit
and some
leafy greenies.

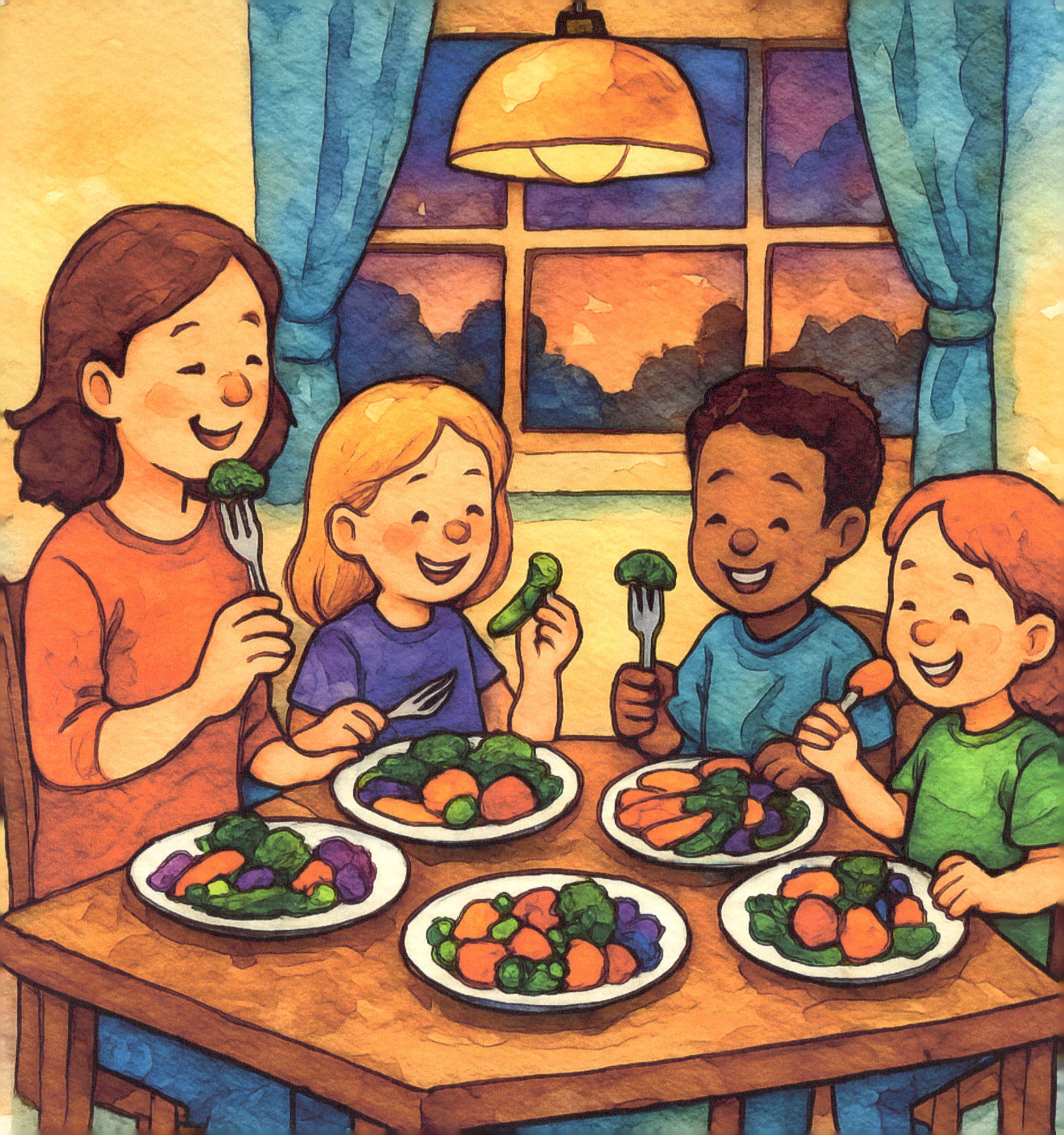

Squash,
peppers,
broccoli,
and cauliflowers-
I could eat them
for hours and hours.

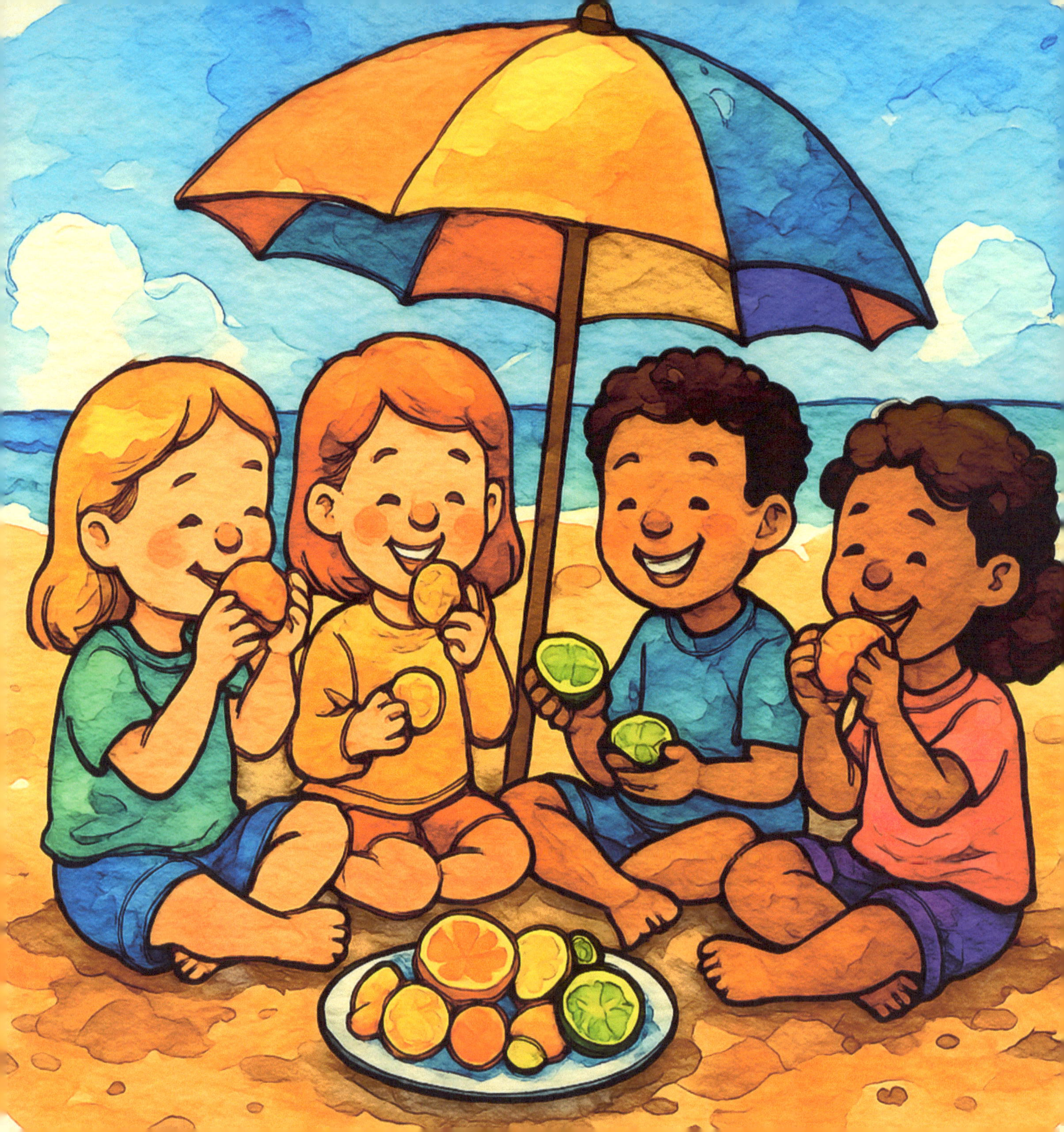

Apricots,
peaches,
lemons,
and limes-
I could eat them
at all times.

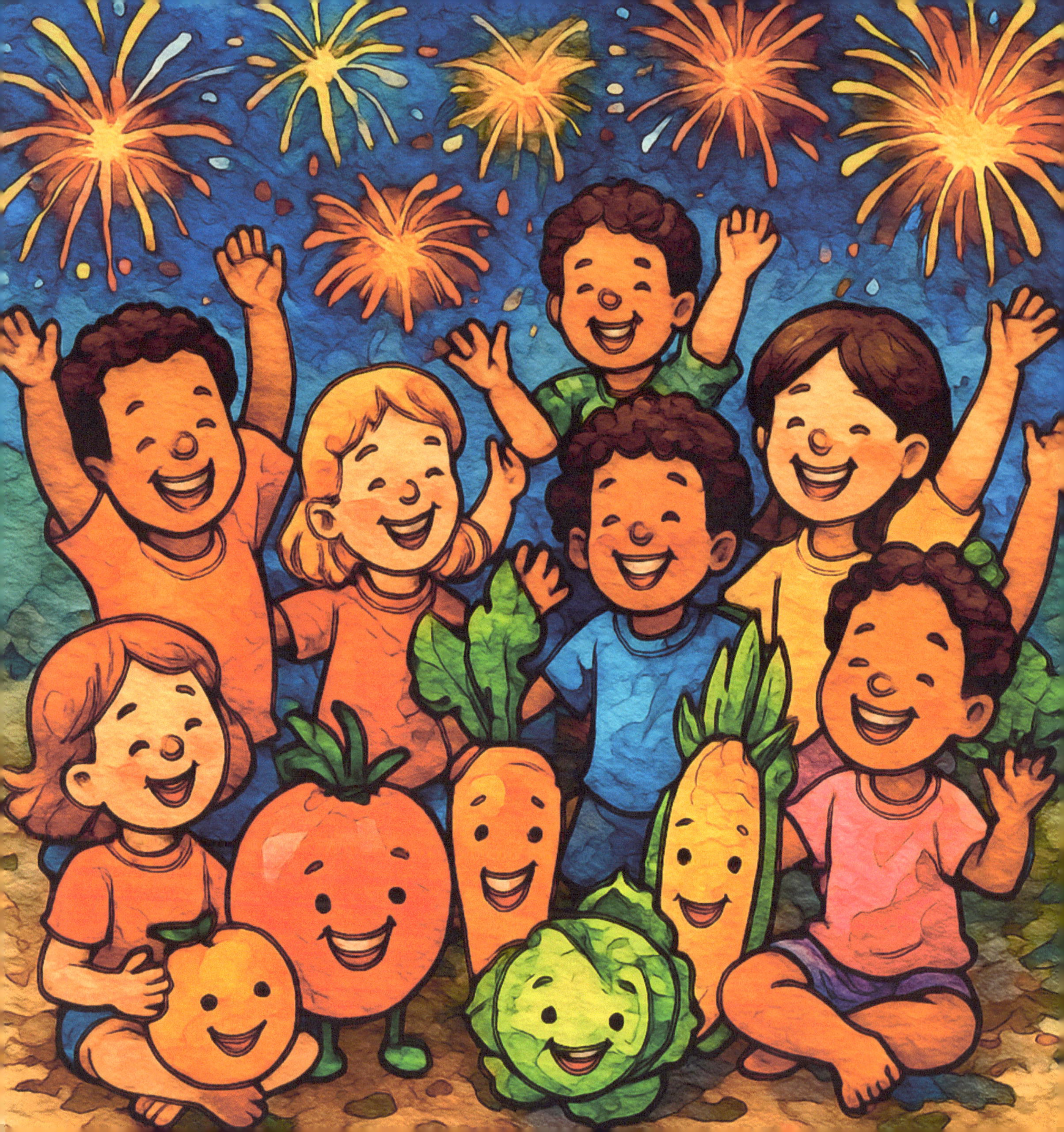

I want to Chomp.

I want to Chew.
Fruits and veggies
are good for you.

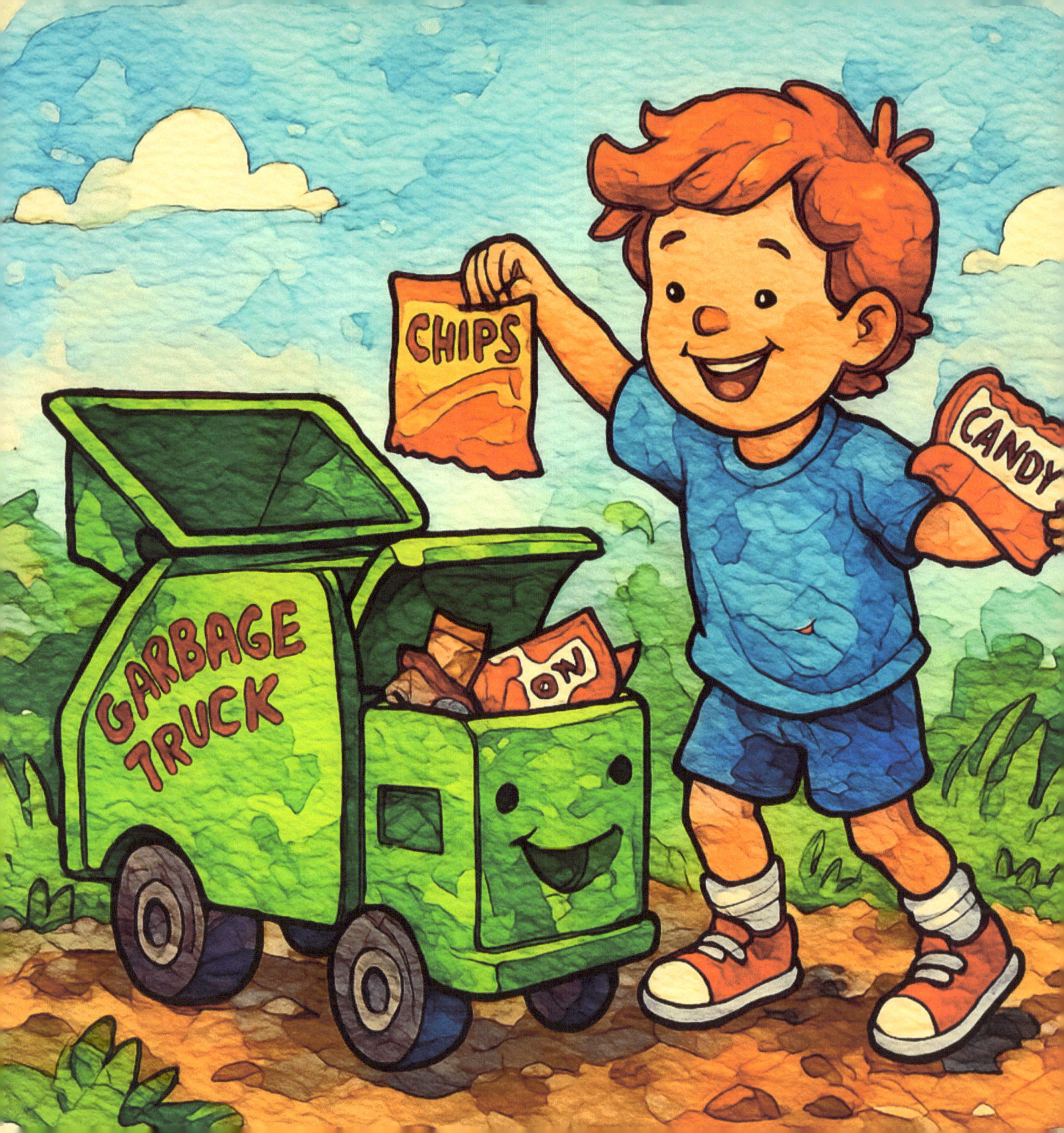

CHIPS
CANDY
GARBAGE TRUCK
OW

Junk food is so
yucky, kucky.
I think I'll put mine in the
garbage truckie.
Where should I start?
What should I do?
I think I know
what I'm going to do.

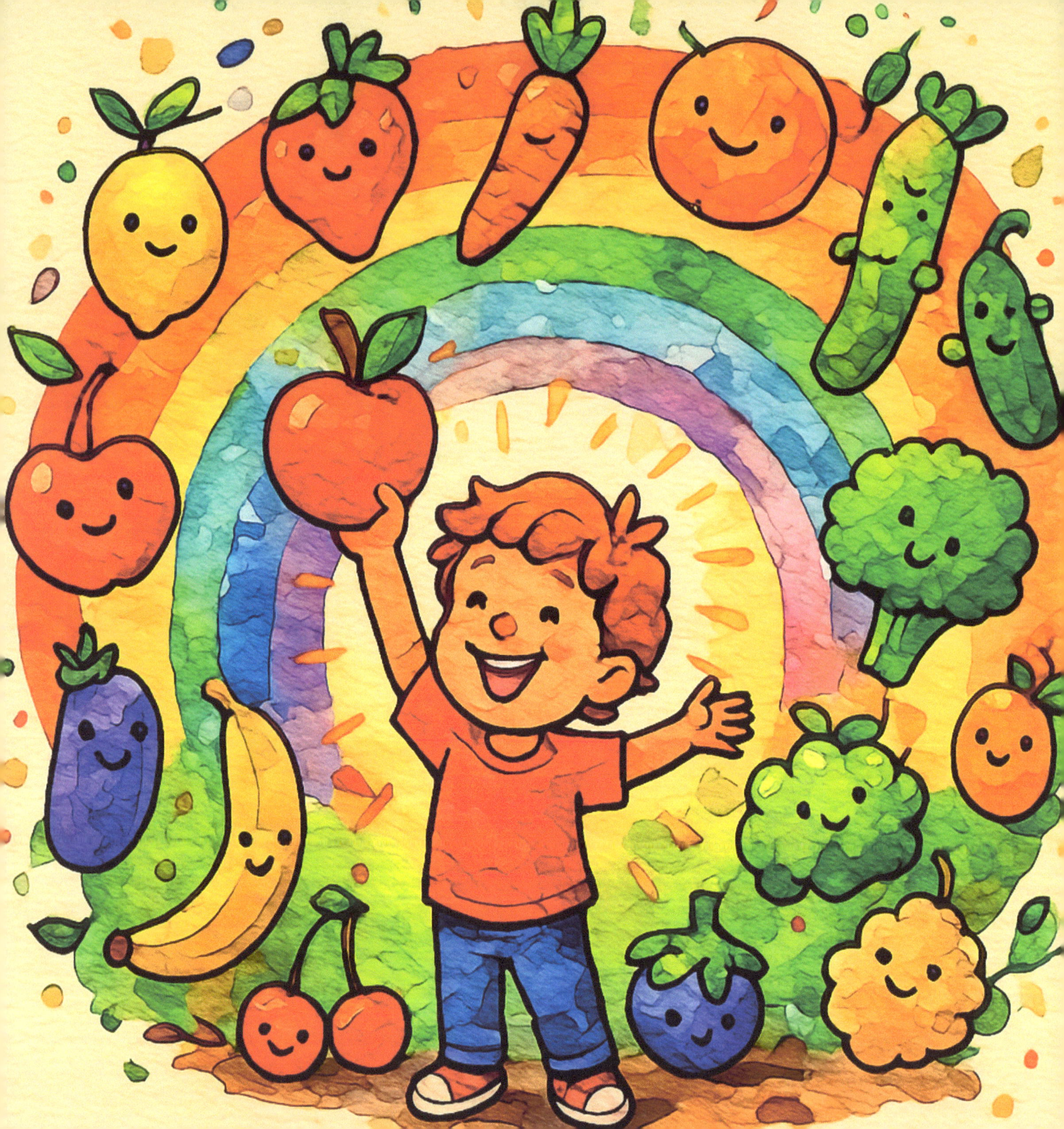

I'm going to Chomp,
and I'm going to Chew.

Why, you may ask?
Because fruits
and veggies
are good for you.